THE PI$$ED OF MIDWIFE'S GUIDE TO HAVING A BABY

WHAT EVERY PARENT SHOULD KNOW

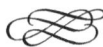

E. BALI

Copyright © 2020 by E. Bali

All rights reserved.

No part of this book may be reproduced in any form or by any electronic or mechanical means, including information storage and retrieval systems, without written permission from the author, except for the use of brief quotations in a book review.

This book is for informational purposes only. Please consult with your health care provider before making any decisions about your or your baby's health.

CONTENTS

Blue Moon Rising Publishing   v
Introduction   vii

1. 1: Pregnancy   1
2. 2: Model of Care   7
3. 3: Public v Private   11
4. 4: What you REALLY need   13
5. 5: Preparing for Labor   17
6. 6: Labour   22
7. 7: Induction of Labor   31
8. 8: Tears to your lady parts   34
9. 9: HOT TIPS For labor   37
10. 10: Pain Relief   40
11. 11: Instrumental Birth   43
12. 12: Emergency Caesarean   45
13. 13: Elective Caesarean   49
14. 14: Your body post birth   53
15. 15: The Fourth Trimester   61
16. 16: Baby's first needles   63
17. 17: Breastfeeding   66
18. 18: Breastfeeding Troubles   71
19. 19: Supplementing   78
20. 20: The first 24 hours   82
21. 21: Visitors + a word about COVD-19   86
22. 22: 24-48 hours   89
23. 23: 48-72 hours   92
24. 24: 96 hours+   95
25. 25: The first six weeks   97
26. 26: Follow up   100
27. 27: Being at home   103

28. 28: Your next baby	105
29. 29: The most important TIPS	107
Afterword	109

BLUE MOON RISING PUBLISHING

THE PI$ED OFF MIDWIFE'S GUIDE TO HAVING A BABY

by E. Bali

INTRODUCTION

After more than a decade working and studying midwifery, I know that new mums need to absorb a lot of information about giving birth to and looking after a sparkly new tiny human.

I also know that no one has the time to sit down and read hundreds of pages on the subject.

Midwives love to teach. We love to empower parents with the right information so that they can look after themselves and their family confidently and safely.

In reality, a woman might stay a day or two in hospital, they might not want to sit through hours of antenatal classes or they might be too pricey. None of these are ideal! I'm "pissed off" because I'm hurrying around the maternity ward, wishing I could give more of my time to deserving families but am often not able to.

INTRODUCTION

In a perfect world I could transfer everything I know right from my brain to yours. So, this is my attempt to do just that!

I present to you, a no nonsense guide to having a baby. Because none of us have time these days, it will be in dot points. It's going to be short, sweet and to the point. This is everything I would ideally tell/teach my patients and their families when I see them, whether it be in antenatal clinic, the birthing suite or postnatal/maternity ward, in one compact place.

These are things that midwives want you to—nay, need you to know. I've also added in links to videos and other good quality resources. I want you to be able to flip through this and get your information quickly. I have no intention of wasting your time.

Check it out while you're still pregnant. Be prepared with information and you'll find you have a less stressful journey because you'll understand what's going on and why. But even if you've already given birth, you'll still find what's presented here to be helpful.

This book is focused on the end of pregnancy, birth and the postnatal phase, so you'll find only a very short section on general pregnancy information.

All the best on your parenting journey

INTRODUCTION

****Everything presented in this book is for informational purposes only. ALWAYS consult your GP/ Obstetrician / Paediatrician/ Midwife/ Psychologist before applying anything you see here or on the internet or ANYWHERE.****

1: PREGNANCY

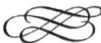

The Health of your baby

- **Your baby's movements are the first sign of well-being**
- From 16 weeks you'll start to notice movements. Keep an eye on these and get familiar with your baby's personality.
- **Do not buy a Doppler. I repeat. Do not buy a Doppler.** (This is the thing that the doctor/midwife uses to listen to the baby's heartbeat). **WHY? Because it is not an indicator of whether a baby is well.** A Doppler only tells you the baby has a heartbeat, not that they are well or unwell. It cannot and should not be used as reassurance. Midwives just do it at appointments because it's exciting for the parents to hear. It should not be used to reassure you if you are worried. Your baby's movements are more important.

- The best way to tell if you should be worried about your baby is how normal their movements are for that time of day. **If your baby's movements are less than they usually are you MUST call your doctor/midwife/hospital immediately for monitoring.**

The health of your mind

- Why don't we talk about this more?
- Make some time **each day** to talk to your baby or read to them (they start to pick up words and emotions from super early on, believe it or not)
- Your baby learns about the world it is about to enter from you. Babies born to super anxious mothers are more anxious themselves. Make time to do some deep breathing, tell your baby they are safe (out loud or inside your head) and tell them you love them.
- Have your partner connect with the baby as well by talking to them. (If your partner is a male, babies love male voices because they can hear the deeper voice more easily inside there).
- Take some time to think about your role as a mother and how you are going through into the new phase of your life.
- Connect to whatever spiritual beliefs you have about birth and life
- If things start to get stressful, hormonal, sad or

angry, take a time out and feel those emotions, don't ignore your feelings or bury them. And then count the things in life you are grateful for. There are some seriously interesting research studies on the effect of 'gratitude' on the body and mind.
- Develop a plan for how to deal with stress, anger, lack of sleep, baby blues and how to make time for self care after the birth.
- Take time for self care weekly (if not daily!)
- Self-care are things that bring you true joy and happiness
- Self care is also attending to the needs of your body and mind, even if it's a chore to do it

Nutrition

- It goes without saying: half or more of your diet should come from fruits and vegetables
- The rest should be meat, diary and carbohydrates (**emerging research is showing diets higher in sugars and unhealthy fats can lead to behavioural problems in children**).
- Those with dietary preferences should check with their doctor for vitamin deficiency
- I.e.: Vegetarians and vegans need to consider their Iron and B12 levels.
- Iron deficiency in pregnancy is very common in even in non vegetarians
- **2L of water a day no excuses**
- Towards the end of pregnancy some women

can get constipated, so up your fibre and water or you can get gentle laxatives from the supermarket. You'll need these for after the birth, anyway.
- Vitamins
- A prenatal vitamin
- + Any extras your doctor advises you: Iron, B12, Vitamin D are common
- The no-go zone:
- Undercooked meat and eggs
- Soft cheese and unpasteurised diary
- Raw fish, cold meats (risk of bacteria like salmonella)
- Big fishes (too much mercury)- shark, tuna
- Organ meats (too much vitamin A can be toxic to babies)
- Alcohol (there is no known 'safe' amount of alcohol we can recommend for pregnancy. The research is saying it is best not to drink at all).

Exercise

- Stay consistent with exercise from pre-pregnancy. Don't go adding new and elaborate things. You might have to tone it down during the end of pregnancy
- Do you **pelvic floor exercises** pronto! (If you want a good sex life after the baby or just want to prevent bladder leakage DO THEM). This is a great video explaining the whole thing:

https://www.youtube.com/watch?v=OArrUPQqCHM

Sleeping

- **Lie on your side from 20 weeks, never on your back.** (Why? Because the blood vessel that supply the baby with oxygen is right down the centre of your body behind the uterus. Every time you lie on your back ,the baby's weight presses on this vessel blocking their own blood flow)
- If you have trouble sleeping by a body pillow or pregnancy pillow. These can be a life saver for finding a good position
- If, towards the end of pregnancy, you are getting a lot of painful Braxton Hicks contractions, it's usually a sign that you need to hydrate and take a rest.
- Swelling
- Puffy feet are normal in pregnancy, especially towards the end. Elevate your feet a couple of times a day to let the fluid drain back. Lie on your side and prop your feet on a couple of cushions.)
- We don't want to see a puffy face or balloon like feet and hands. Make sure you get your blood pressure and urine checked if you notice a large amount of swelling.

Vaccinations in pregnancy

- **Flu Vaccine**- WHY? Catching influenza in pregnancy or afterwards can land you and your baby in ICU. Not worth the risk
- Boostrix (Tetanus, Diphtheria **Whooping cough**)- needed for the whooping cough part as your baby is vulnerable to get it from birth and we can't vaccinate newborns so we vaccinate the mother so they can get immunity through you and your breastmilk.

<u>Things to flag immediately (day or night) with your doctor or midwife:</u>

- Constant severe headaches
- Blurred vision/stars in eyes randomly
- Extremely itchy palms
- Severe rashes
- Vaginal bleeding
- Constant leaking of watery fluid from vagina
- Baby is moving less than usual for the time of day
- If you have a strange sensation of 'not feeling pregnant anymore'
- If you feel something is not right or that something is wrong
- If you just don't feel well.

2: MODEL OF CARE

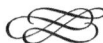

There are a few different ways of getting your pregnancy care. Funnily enough, not many people are aware of all the choices.

The gold standard of care remains to be that whoever you choose for your care, they should be **constant/the same the whole way through**. Ideally the person who delivers your baby is someone who knows you and your health well.

More recently, due to consumer demand for cost friendly choices, new models of care have propped up. The new models we have seen are group obstetrics and private team midwifery/obstetrics. I'll explain these below.

Public Antenatal Clinic

- Through your hospital, you'll see a mixture of midwives and doctors for each appointment. Usually covered by public health funding.

GP shared care

- This is where your GP is certified to give antenatal care. Most of your visits will be with this doctor with one or two pregnancy checks with a hospital Obstetrician and/or Midwife.

Midwifery Group Practice (usually birth centre model)

- Through a hospital. A midwife from the group will see you at each appointment so that you meet each one of the team. Then one of them will be on call every day to take private phone calls and then look after you in labor.
- If they operate through a birth centre it usually a separate part of the hospital or in a different building completely. They specialise in natural pain relief methods and low-risk women. They might even do home-births.
- If you are looking for an epidural during labor, your care is usually transferred back to hospital midwives.
- They do home visits after birth up to 6 weeks

Private Midwifery

- A single private midwife cares for you antenatally, during labor/birth and does home visits after birth too
- They can prescribe medication
- Often do home births or have an agreement with a hospital to use one of their rooms.

Private Obstetrician

A private doctor who is also surgeon specialising in abnormal pregnancy and caesarean section.

They also take on women having healthy pregnancies (who might for example wish to have a caesarean or are anxious about having complications)

Advised for high-risk pregnancies

Group Obstetrician care

- Newer model where a team of obstetricians provide your care lowering the cost overall
- You might meet a different obstetrician at each appointment and not know who is on call the night of your birth

Team Private obstetrics + Private midwifery

- A team of private midwives who work together with a private Obstetrician or two who share the appointments. The Midwives will look after you in labor and the obstetrician does any required surgery + midwifery visits 6 weeks post birth.
- You get the benefits of knowing a smaller team of professionals.
- Very popular mode

Fun fact The biggest maternity hospitals worldwide:

Southern Hemisphere: The Mater Mothers Hospital Brisbane= 10,000/year

Europe: The National Hospital Dublin = 10,000 /year

US: Northside Hospital Atlanta= 27,000/year

Africa: Punwani Maternity Hospital Nairobi= 27,000/year

In the World: Fabella Hospital Manila= 60-100 per day (approx 30,000/year)

3: PUBLIC V PRIVATE

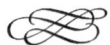

There are pros and cons to both. The key for you is to decide which will suit your family and your budget. Private Health insurance is getting quite expensive, so make sure you shop around and see what options are available in your area.

Private

- $$$
- Single specialist care provider for whole pregnancy and birth
- Midwifery care during labour, obstetrician comes in and out and catches the baby at the end or does interventions for the birth.
- Longer length of stay in hospital often with hotel options (often 4-6 days)
- Better food
- Nicer rooms

- Small out of pocket

Public

- Often no or very little cost (e.g. partner meals, take home medications, extra services.)
- Possibly different doctors/midwives seeing you each appointment
- Midwifery group practice option available for low risk mothers
- Midwifery care during labour, doctors enter room if review needed or for concerns
- Short length of stay in hospital (anywhere from 6 hours to 3 days for caesarean)

4: WHAT YOU REALLY NEED

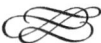

BABY

The obvious big guns:

- Cot
- Car seat
- Pram
- Bassinet (not essential but makes life easier to begin with)

Baby Clothes

- Jumpsuits with full arms and legs inbuilt mittens. (If your baby is going to be on the smaller side, less than 3kg, I recommend getting the terry-towling kind. I've found babies keep warm in this much better. But big babies over 4kg tend to overheat in them.)

- Jumpsuits with short sleeves/no legs (especially for summer babies in hot climates)
- Jumpers and woollen clothes for babies in cold climates
- Singlets (especially for the first weeks and for smaller babies)
- Beanies (for outside in cool weather only + the first 24 hours of life)
- Socks or booties (especially if small, otherwise optional).
- Large muslin wraps (lots)
- Thicker blankets for on top
- Sleeping bags (for later weeks, they don't work to settle babies in the first few days)

*Babies are messy. You will get wee, poo, vomit and milk everywhere, so get plenty of everything.

*A note on sizing. Over the years I have observed baby clothes to be getting bigger. I don't know if this objectively true, but in the last three years I have noticed parents complaining that their newborn size (0000) is way too big. So I would recommend that if you know your baby is average sized and definitely if smaller or you are Indian/Asian descent, get 00000s (prem size) so you have clothes that fit for the first 2-3weeks. Note that babies lose weight after birth before they start to gain.

The things you don't need for Baby

- Cot bumpers (not SIDS safe- can suffocate the baby if they roll and can't move)
- Inside beanies (beanies are not SIDS safe for sleeping and a healthy baby should not need a beanie on inside after the first days of life)
- Mittens (they simply won't stay on and I dare you to try. The best sort are the ones that are in built with jumpsuits- they fold over the hands.)

Things for breastfeeding Mums:

- Nipple cream
- Hydrogel nipple pads or bamboo (everyone has a different preference)
- Breastfeeding pillow
- Breastpump (the Spectra if it is in your price range otherwise you can hire or buy a medela/avent brand second hand. Always get electric.)
- A Haka pump can also be useful (while you breastfeed on one side, the other side can leak- so you can pop on the Haka on the unused side to collect extras). But this is not essential.
- Bottles & teats
- Steriliser (optional because you can do the old-fashioned submerge in boiling water for 10 mins)

- Breastfeeding bra
- Breastfeeding friendly tops
- * I would say that having a tin of formula in the pantry is a good idea in case of emergency in the middle of the night.

∽

Things for MUM in general

- Belly bands/recovery shorts
- Maternity pads (you'd be surprised how many people forget these)
- And/ Or Absorbent undies (from the pharmacy- women LOVE these, less messy, no laundry.)
- Appropriate regular undies (if you have a Caesarean you don't want the band sitting on your wound- so get super big ones or super small ones)
- Laxatives
- Perineal Squirting bottle (If you have a vaginal birth, urinating post birth can be uncomfortable, so having fresh water flushing your 'bits' while you wee can make it feel much nice. Plus, if you have stitches, this can help clean those more easily.)
- Painkillers you should have at home: Paracetamol/Tylenol, Ibuprofen/ Diclofenac (after birth only, not allowed in pregnancy)

5: PREPARING FOR LABOR

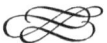

- Do not tell people your **due date**. You'll regret it if you go over. People will keep messaging you with "when's the baby coming?" and you'll get either annoyed or anxious or both.
- Instead, when people ask your due date, tell them the due month instead. If anything tell them later rather than sooner. (If you're due at the end of September, tell them October instead)
- Everyone has been brainwashed, your due date is not when you are due, it is simply when you are 40 weeks. Every woman's body gives birth differently and between 37-42 weeks is considered normal.
- **Walk**
- Adjust your pre-pregnancy level of exercise to a manageable level, but do not stop. Labor is a

marathon and you need your energy and stamina to get through to end
- **Sleep**
- As much as you need to keep active, your body also needs rest as it is providing for two people. Be kind to yourself.
- Sit on an exercise ball rather than a normal chair
- **Don't make a habit of 'leaning back positions'** try to be on your side or forward leaning as much as possible (to avoid "back-to-back labor" where the baby's spine is facing your spine- makes for a painful back labor)
- **Eat dates** (a couple of small studies found some correlation between eating dates and benefits in labor and birth) https://evidencebasedbirth.com/evidence-eating-dates-to-start-labor/
- **Perineal massage from 34 weeks** to reduce the probability of tearing. This is where you massage your vagina and stretch it gently. Instructions here: https://www.youtube.com/watch?v=Wm2aqVOG6Tc
- Get rid of your pubic hair
- This is always down to personal preference of course but hair can make things a lot messier during and especially after birth. If you're wanting to keep stitches clean afterwards, not having hair is beneficial.
- If you don't want to wax/laser etc, keep it short and your midwives will thank you. (I have seen

clamps stuck on long pubic hair before, it's not pleasant!)
- Note: midwives/doctors don't mind too much about whether you have hair down there or not, while it can make things less messy for us, this is for your benefit/comfort.
- Consider **antenatal expressing**- ask your care provider for details. This is where you collect milk from your breasts, now, for after birth. You won't get much to start with but it'll increase and you'll thank yourself when you have a hungry baby in your arms. Once you learn the technique, you collect the colostrum in little syringes and freeze them. You can start at 36-37 weeks as it can stimulate labor to start. The more you empty from your breasts, the more they produce.
- **Talk with your partne**r about:
- How you will manage stress, lack of sleep and low moods when you get home. You'll feel some strong emotions, positive and negative, so you may as well be prepared for them.
- Everyone has different set levels for their mood. Baby blues will hit you day 3 post birth. A low mood can persist and evolve into depression and/or anxiety. If mental health issues like anxiety and depression are already factors in your life, you need to have a plan for how to deal with it in hospital and once your home. Things like;
- Knowing each other's triggers

- Knowing when each person needs space and when they don't
- Knowing what each person needs in the relationship and how you both will compromise when the baby come
- Knowing what each person needs to feel loved and fulfilled
- Knowing what each person needs for their self care routine
- Promise to be flexible and communicate needs and issues
- How you will manage visitors, particularly the role of the grandparents and **where your boundaries are**.
- How you will manage food and cleaning of the house and care of any pets
- How your partner will mange their work/business commitments
- Pay attention to your body
- Don't ignore when you are thirsty, hungry or tired (mentally and physically)
- Read/Watch
- Learn different positions for labor/birth
- Learn your pain relief options
- Evidenced based birth website
- Australian Birth podcast/ relevant to your country— this helps develop realistic expectations of your birth.
- The business of being born documentary
- Learn CPR and infant resuscitation/ First Aid.

If you're going to be a parent, you should know this.

6: LABOUR

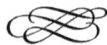

- You have been brainwashed- labor is not like the movies
- People always have the need to tell you the worst birth stories. ("MY birth was 50 hours long".... etc).
- Listen to your mother and her birth stories. Watch one born every minute or listen to Australian Birth podcast. Listen to **real stories** and a lot of them.
- Some people don't want to do this, which is fine. I would only advise you to ask your health care provider questions, and/or read reliable information (ahem. Below).

Labor is the process of your **cervix** (entrance to the uterus, at the end of your vagina) softening and opening until it's disappeared. When you are fully dilated, your cervix can't be felt anymore.

There are **4 stages** of labor:

Stage 1 is where you go from 0cm (**closed**) to 10cm dilation (**fully** dilated) and we split this into two parts.

- In order for your cervix to dilate, you need strong, regular and painful contractions.
- **<u>Early labour is from 0-3cm</u>**
- This phase can take many hours and is best done at home.
- The contractions can be painful but are often irregular or far apart.
- In a ten-minute period you'll get between 1 and 3 contractions and will differ in how strong they are.
- The contractions at this stage stay the same. Once the contractions are progressively getting stronger and longer, it's time to 'call the midwife'.
- Most people are best doing this part at home as long as pregnancy has been healthy and without risk factors.
- **<u>Active labor is from 3-10cm</u>**
- This is where you're getting down and dirty
- You'll have 3-4 contractions in ten minutes
- Importantly, you feel the contractions becoming MORE painful, longer and more regular. That's how you tell the difference

between active and early labor. In active labour your contractions are progressing.

Contractions

- **Braxton-Hicks** (practice contractions you can get from 34 weeks) feel like your tummy is going super tight. Some people describe it as like a vice around the stomach. Baby might notice these and wriggle around a lot when it happens. The more of these practice contractions you get the better- your body is preparing for labour!
- Feel like period pains at first, and then it feels like a stretching/pulling sensation down low in your pelvis. This sensation means that your cervix is trying to open up. You also feel that tightness all around your stomach.
- Contractions come in waves. They start, build up, then build back down. You'll get a rest for a minute or two, then the next one starts back up. Use these rest periods wisely.
- Midwives will feel these contractions by gently touching the top of your stomach. You uterus is a muscle and goes hard when its contracting (like any other muscle) so midwives can feel a contraction coming even before you do. When they are touching your stomach they are feeling how strong and long the contractions

are. This is part of their midwifery assessment of your labor.

The **2nd stage** of labour is from fully dilated (10cm) to the birth of your baby.

- In this stage your baby is moving through the vagina/birth canal, through your uterus contracting and pushing
- Most women without an epidural will start involuntarily pushing. This is where your body will seem as if its pushing on its own. And if you tell a woman to stop, most of the time they will tell you they can't.
- If you have an epidural, your midwife/doctor will tell you when to push. They'll tell you when a contraction is happening and advise you on when to start and stop pushing.

Transition

- The most important thing I can tell you here is what is called **transition**. This is where your body is getting ready to go into the second stage and can start from 7cm onwards. For some reason, if you don't have an epidural, women feel scared, like they can't do it and start asking for help/to get the baby out.
- If a woman in a labor says to me "I can't do this anymore" or "I'm scared." I'm going to suspect she's transitional. It is really important to know

that this stage exists, and that it'll happen, so that when you're going through it, you know the end is approaching and you're almost there. **I can't count the number of epidurals put in only to have the baby be born minutes later because the woman did not know about transition.**

- **Once you are fully dilated you can expect your baby to be born within the next 2-2.5 hours.**
- It is also really hard to convince someone about this when they are in labor, so congratulations on knowing about this in advance, because it'll make your life a lot easier.

Birth

- So the hardest part of this stage is getting to see the baby's head. It's a two steps forward, one step back situation. The baby's head moves back and forth until finally, he's sitting so down low that he won't move backwards.
- If you don't have an epidural, this is where women start to feel the 'burning' sensation in the vagina. So Hot tip: request hot compresses on your vagina during this time. Studies show that it aids in stretching pain and helps prevent tears.
- Once the baby's head is born, he'll be looking downwards. Then he needs to turn and look sideways (either left or right) to give birth to

- the top shoulder, then the bottom shoulder, and then he's out!
- The baby should go straight onto your naked chest for skin-skin and bonding time. He needs to know you are there, plus it helps regulate his temperature, breathing and heart rate.
- The midwives will dry him thoroughly so he doesn't get cold and check him out to make sure he doing all the right things.
- They should only remove him if they are worried: If after one minute of life he is not breathing, has a poor heart rate and looking floppy, he should be taken to the resus cot for some breaths of air. Most babies respond to this very quickly if they're a bit 'stunned' from birth and rarely they need CPR to get them going.
- So at this stage usually the baby should still be connected to you via his cord. **Best practice is to let this cord pulse until all the blood from the placenta is back into the baby which can take a few minutes**. This stage should not be interrupted unless the baby needs resuscitation, where the cord **must be** clamped and cut early.

The 3rd stage of birth is from the birth of the baby to the birth of the placenta.

- You thought it was all over? Nup! One last

thing, the great unifier of mother and baby, the placenta has to be delivered.
- Lucky for you, there are no bones in the placenta, so it sort of just slides out nicely.
- After the baby is born your uterus needs to do one powerful contraction. Then, the placenta slides off the wall of the uterus and sits there ready to be pushed/pulled out.
- Ideally, once the cord stops pulsing, the baby's cord is clamped with a yellow plastic clamp, and then cut to separate.
- There are two ways to deal with this part:
- **Passive management:** This is where we do nothing, we just wait for the placenta to separate and you push it out on your own. You must be at low risk of haemorrhage to do this type.
- **Active management:** The second biggest cause of maternal death in birth worldwide is haemorrhage post birth (too much bleeding). So most midwives/doctors will advise you to do it this way. After birth, the midwife will give you an injection into your leg. This medication is called oxytocin and is what makes your uterus contract. After a few minutes, your doctor/midwife will then gently pull on the cord to help it come out.
- Ask to look at your placenta afterwards, you won't get the chance again and it's super interesting to see one of your organs outside of your body (that could be just the midwife in

me though). If mums aren't interested in this, often dads are. Have a look! Your body is amazing.
- The hospital can then dispose of the placenta as medical waste or you can take it home.
- Some cultures bury the placenta
- Some people give the placenta to a service that dries it and makes them into tablets to take. The research behind this is still preliminary but there is a small amount of evidence to suggest that it can prevent postnatal depression.

The 4th Stage of Birth

- This is the sacred hours after birth
- Its super important for both mother and baby to have an uninterrupted time skin to skin for the first hour after birth.
- This so beneficial for not only the physical well-being of both, but the mental well-being too.
- Babies are happier and better off with mum
- Weighing and needles can wait an hour, seriously. If anyone is trying to rush you (and both of you are well) it is unwarranted.

Birth plans

- The best plan is a flexible one. Having a rigid

birth plan with no room to move, never works, especially in hospital.
- I promise you, that nurses/midwives/doctors go to work wanting to make a positive difference in people's lives. They are not out to get you unlike what popular opinion would have you think.
- You are meant to work with your health care provider, it is not a "you do what I say" relationship.
- If you have a very fixed idea of what your vaginal birth should be like, I would look into having a private midwife for your pregnancy and birth care.
- You should have an idea of what music you want and what pain relief you would like/not like, and who you want in the room with you.
- You should discuss your plan with your health care provider/hospital because the amount of misinformed birth plans I have seen is phenomenal.

NOTE: After your first baby, as a general rule, you can expect to half your length of labor. It's much easier the second/third etc time. After the second baby all these stages of labor can cross over and happen together.

When they ALL happen at the same time, that's when the baby is born "en caul" meaning, baby, placenta and waters (waters not broken) all come out at the same time!

7: INDUCTION OF LABOR

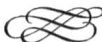

An Induction of labour is where you are artificially putting your body into labour rather than waiting for it to start on its own.

There are many reasons for this:

- Social reasons: An elective induction is where there is no medical reason for the baby to be born early, but the parents have requested it. This is to be avoided where possible.
- Medical reasons: Basically your health care provider has determined that given the evidence, your baby's health is better off on the outside than in the uterus.

Inducing your labor means breaking your waters and getting your contractions going with a hormone drip.

In order to break your waters, your cervix needs to be 'ripe'. This means its feeling soft and open enough that we can pop the membranes.

If your cervix is not ready for labor (often for your first baby before 40 weeks pregnancy), one of three things can be used to help with this:

- Prostaglandin (Prostin): A gel that is inserted under the cervix to soften and ripen the cervix.
- Cervidil: a vaginal pessary (tablet) that is placed under the cervix. It slowly releases a hormone to soften and ripen the cervix
- Cervical Balloon: Actually two balloons. These are small balloons inflated either side of the cervix to place gentle pressure on them, causing them to trigger ripening.

After your cervix is a little open: (1cm is enough)

- Your midwife or doctor with break your waters with a small hook (you won't feel this) and then start the hormone drip (**Oxytocin**: trade names: Pitocin & Syntocinon).
- Every half hour/hour your midwife will put your drip up until your contractions are 3-4 in ten minutes and getting stronger.
- This drip will be regulated up/down by your

midwife so you don't have too many/too little contractions.
- The CTG- this monitor will be strapped to you periodically during your induction and throughout your entire labor.

CTG:

- It shows the baby's heart rate variability (a pattern of beat to beat electrical signals) that tells us if enough oxygen is getting to the baby's brain.
- The frequency of contractions
- It is important to not place too much of your attention on the CTG- let your midwife/doctor assess it
- The baby's heart rate will change over the course of labor, some of these changes are normal in response to contractions and the stresses of labor.
- These machines tell us how likely the baby is to be compromised. Midwives and doctors grade the trace every half an hour at least.
- It is important to note that they are not 100% accurate and have a high 'false positive rate' meaning that the trace might show concerning patterns when the baby has enough oxygen. However, because these traces are the only industry standard measurements of baby's wellbeing in labour/induction, your health care provider **must** act on what they see.

8: TEARS TO YOUR LADY PARTS

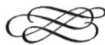

Yes, your vagina and/ or perineum (the space between your anus and vagina) MAY tear.

- In most first time mums it usually does a little
- This part of your body is **made** to tear and heal well
- Asian & Indian women are known to be more likely to tear. So please you ladies take heed.

Types of tears:

- 1st degree/ graze: shallow tear to the skin only
- 2nd degree- tear to the muscle - also common, needs stitches
- 3rd degree- deeper tears to their anus (not as common), needs stitches in theatre and physio follow up.
- Other tears: clitoral and urethral (more

common un upright, forward leaning pushing positions).
- **Episiotomy**: is where your doctor or midwife cuts your perineum usually because it looks this is the safest way for you to tear. We direct the 'tear' away from your anus, as natural tears can go straight down there. Sometimes an episiotomy stops worse tears from happening. You are given local anaesthetic before this happens. But often by the time the baby's head is stretching here, your sensation is very altered.
- **You'll be stitched up after birth with dissolvable stitches that'll take 7-10 days to dissolve**

A few things prevent it:

- **Perineal massage** & stretching in pregnancy
- **Pelvic floor/ Kegel exercises**. DO THEM. When you brush your teeth. DO THEM. I know women who have had 6 babies and their pelvic floors were fine, and why? Because they did their exercises. If you don't do this, you can wee and poo when you don't mean to (before as well as after birth). DO THEM.
- Heat packs during second stage (pushing stage)
- Extra credit: You can buy devices (eg "epi-no") that are like balloons that stretch your vagina bit by bit. You have full control over this and it is evidence based.

How to deal with a tear

- Keep it clean (wash it twice a day + when you poo).
- Ice it for min 3 days (hospitals have special ice packs for this: aka a frozen condom)
- It'll sting when you urinate so wee in the shower + flush with water while you wee (you can buy a squirty bottle for this) and it'll feel so much better.
- Make sure your stitches are checked daily while in hospital

9: HOT TIPS FOR LABOR

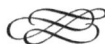

- Labor is controlled by a tens of thousands of years old part of our brain. It should be treated with respect.
- The part of your brain that controls labor is inhibited by the newer part (neocortex). So excessive thinking and analysing interferes with this. Give in to your inner animal!
- Bright lights and adrenaline also interfere with labouring hormones
- Adrenaline directly opposes oxytocin (labouring hormone) so keeping things calm and relaxed is super important to keep contractions happening.
- Stay hydrated
- Eat lightly

Having a baby on your back is unnatural. Have you ever seen an animal give birth lying on their back? No, they either go lay their side or stand and squat. There are two reasons for this:

- Gravity
- Your pelvis is actually wider by 0.5-1cm (which can be significant in a small space) in a squatting position then lying down. Your baby needs room to make the adjustments required to come out.
- Move around, lean forward, lie on your side. Be active, moving your pelvis around will help your baby move down and into a good position.

<u>Try different positions</u>. There are SO many positions to try in both the first stage and the pushing stage.

- 1st stage: Side lying, peanut cushion (helps keep your legs open on your side), birth ball, forward leaning over top of bed or on birth mat, hands and knees, standing/swaying supported by birth partner.
- 2nd stage (pushing phase): Birth stool, Squat bar, hands and knees, standing, side lying with top leg supported (using the birthing bed)
- 3rd stage (placenta): on toilet, squatting or lying back
- Just google 'birth positions' so you can see what's available.
- **The key here is knowing your options beforehand.** It makes it much easier in the

moment if you already know what you like and what will feel good. Then when your baby is trying to tell you to move a certain way, you'll know how to go about doing that.
- Always trust your instincts, being in certain positions will help the baby move a certain way as they descend into your pelvis.
- Modern birthing rooms have all the necessary equipment to help you do any of these positions.

Reasons you should alert your midwife/ doctor:

- You break your waters (note the colour and how much, pink and clear are great, green or brown need to be noted)
- Baby's movements are not normal for time of day
- You feel unwell
- Bleeding from your vagina
- You feel like you need to push (bowel pressure- feels like you want to poo badly)
- If you feel like the baby is on the way soon, you should stay at home and call an ambulance.
- Same thing if you are in the car. If you feel that the baby is going to be born the car, pull over and call an ambulance

10: PAIN RELIEF

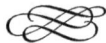

How many times have I had to explain these options to a woman while she was in throes of labor? Countless. Please know these in advance! You have to be able to make a sound decision at the time.

There are two types of pain relief in labor. Medications and non-medicated forms.

Non-medicated:

Shower/Bath

For any time in labor but especially if you're at home

(If you have broken your waters and are at home, you should not take a bath- if you are in hospital and have broken your waters then you can).

Heat packs

On your back and across your pelvis can help provide relief.

TENS Machine

have seen women use this as their only pain relief during labor! Some women love the sensation, others don't. This is a little device connected to sticky straps that sit on your back. They provide little vibrations onto you skin that can dramatically reduce your pain. Especially great for back pain. (There are even little versions that people use for severe period pain. Google: "Livia").

Some women can find the vibrations to be "annoying" or unhelpful. You won't know if you don't try.

They are expensive so most physio departments in hospitals rent them out.

Massage

Gently on your lower back using a bit of oil or moisturiser in small circles can really make reduce back pain.

In certain types of labor pressure like this dosen't help and makes back pain worse.

Medications

Paracetamol

Best taken for early labor when you're at home. Best to try this before other medications. If this takes your pain away, then you're definitely not in labor.

Panadeine Forte/Oxycodone

If you are given the okay by your healthcare provider to take this, then it can definitely help early on.

Cons: Possible nausea and definitely constipation

Nitrous gas and air

Takes the edge of contractions. Can be turned up or down. Does not reach the baby.

Cons: possible nausea, dizzyness.

Pethidine/Morphine

Strong pain relief, relaxing, can get you through transition

Cons: nausea/vomiting/space out feeling/if given too close to birth (1-2 hours) can make baby sleepy upon delivery and more likely to need resuscitation.

Epidural

The ultimate form of pain relief. If it's working well you won't feel pain or temperature from your bump downwards. It also reduces your blood pressure (good if you have hypertension or PET).

Cons: Lowers your blood pressure, can be 'patchy' in effect, can slow your contractions and your whole labor. Increases your chances of having an obstructed labor, a Vaccum/Forceps delivery or Caesarean Section.

11: INSTRUMENTAL BIRTH

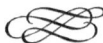

This type of birth is required when the mother is fully dilated, but for some reason (e.g. heavy epidural or exhaustion) the baby is not descending through the birth canal

Baby's head is observed afterwards to check for any changes swelling/blood collection

If an instrumental birth is not successful, a Caesarean section is required.

Vacuum/Ventouse Delivery

- A little suction cup is placed onto the baby's head
- Both mother and doctor put effort in to push and pull
- Only 3-4 pulls allowed
- Episiotomy often needed (sometimes not)

Forceps Delivery

- Used when more effort is required to deliver baby (e.g if mother's pushing has little effect due a heavy epidural)
- They look like salad tongs but cushion the baby's head nicely
- Doctor has more control
- An episiotomy is required
- Will need physiotherapy followup for mother
- Baby can often get small marks or bruises that go away within days

12: EMERGENCY CAESAREAN

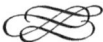

There are emergencies and there are *emergencies*.

To those of us that work in a hospital, an emergency cesarean is one that wasn't planned or anticipated before hand.

If you've gone into hospital/antenatal appointment and they have said to you that you need to have your baby now, and induction is not an option OR this is a decision made during labor

Some common reasons for an Emergency Caesarean:

- Baby becomes distressed (babies are made to cope through labor, however for a number of reasons, they can get tired, or not cope with the contractions or the pressure of the birth canal)
- Dilating too slowly or not at all
- Obstructed labor (the baby is 'stuck')

- Antepartum Haemorrhage (bleeding during pregnancy)
- Severe Pre-eclampsia
- Mother is very unwell

Hospitals categorise emergencies (cat 1 cat 2 cat 3)

- Cat 1- baby needs to be born immediately (within 10mins), reasons include: baby's heart rate goes down and doesn't come back up, cord prolapse (cord coming out first), heavy bleeding)
- Cat 2- baby needs to be born within 30-60 mins
- Cat 3- baby needs to be born within 60-90 mins
- These time frames might differ between hospitals and countries

- Things often move pretty quickly once the decision has been made to go through with a caesarean.
- You'll sign a consent form explaining the risks and benefits
- If you don't already, you'll have a drip put in and be dressed in a theatre gown
- They'll wheel you to theatre on your bed and your partner will be asked to put theatre scrubs on.

- If you don't already and there is time, an anaesthetist will put in a spinal anaesthetic (heavier than an epidural, if you already have an epidural put in, they'll 'top it up').
- If there is no time to wait 10mins for the epidural to be inserted, then a general anaesthetic will be given so the mother will be asleep during delivery. This is not preferred, but only done in absolute emergencies. And in this case, the birthing partner will wait outside and the midwife will bring them the baby straight after birth.

- Once the baby is born, he/she is taken to the baby's team (a midwife and a doctor) for drying, checking over and wrapping. The baby is then usually taken to mum for a cuddle before dad and the baby are taken to another room for weighing and first injections.
- Dad then waits for mum in the recovery room for usually 30-40minutes.
- Once mum joins them in recovery, the midwife can help mum breastfeed if mum is feeling well.
- Mum usually stays in recovery for an hour or so for monitoring, and if all is well, your midwife from the ward will receive you and everyone will be transferred to ward together.
- After transfer to ward both mum and baby will

be monitored very frequently for 4-6 hours, then less frequently after that.
- The urinary catheter (tube in your bladder that collects your wee for you) usually stays in until between 6-24 hours depending on the midwife/doctor assessment and hospital policy and ward culture.
- Mum will stay in bed until advised to get up to walk around and/or shower.
- The midwife will help mum feed and change the baby/teach dad for the first day/night.

13: ELECTIVE CAESAREAN

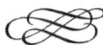

There are many medical reasons why a woman would be advised to have a caesarean section without trying to labor first. The most common:

- Emergency caesarean for their previous baby
- Baby's estimated size is big (with the knowledge that this is an educated guess only)
- Placenta praevia (placenta covers the cervix)
- Breech position (there are not many doctors who will attempt a vaginal breech birth anymore, and if they do, there are strict criteria)
- Severe pre-eclampsia or hypertension
- Poor blood flow to the baby (issues with the placenta)
- Strong mental health history (severe anxiety, PTSD)
- Some women simply choose to have a caesarean because it is their choice. You are

well within your right to choose this, however make sure you understand the risk of mum and baby complications are higher.

Risks:

- Higher risk of haemorrhage, infection, difficulty urinating, severe pain.
- Higher risk of baby needing to go to the nursery for breathing difficulties (usually from fluid in their lungs)
- Higher risk of placental issues *next* pregnancy
- Vaginal births have their risks as well, so it's about weighing up all these and seeing what is right for you. Do not let other people give you their judgements on you for your choice. **It is your body and no one else's business except for your doctor/midwife.**

People always feel the need to give you their opinion. Congratulations, welcome to parenting. You need to learn to be confident and comfortable in the decisions you make about your body and your life. That puts you in good stead to not worry about what other people think.

- An elective caesarean is a pretty calm and controlled process.
- It is usually booked around 38-39 weeks gestation so that there is less of a chance you'll go into labor and have to have it done in the

middle of the night. However, we see this happen a lot. **Babies often have their own plans that they don't tell us about. Go with the flow.**

- You'll be asked to go in a few hours before the operation to get checked in and prepared.
- **HOT TIP**: get your pubic hair waxed or shave your self beforehand. Doing it in hospital is a lot messier and trust me, you want a professional to do that, not a midwife with a hospital grade clipper. The cut is on your lower bikini line area, but the dressing they put on goes a lot lower than that. Be kind to yourself and get rid of your public hair at least from this top area. You'll thank yourself when you go to take your dressing off.
- A Midwife will walk you down to theatre to speak with the nurses and the anaesthetist. This doctor makes sure you are safe during the operation while the obstetrician does the surgery. They also write your pain relief and medications for afterwards.
- (The next section is the same as for emergency caesarean):
- Once the baby is born, he/she is taken to the baby's team (a midwife and a doctor) for drying, checking over and wrapping. The baby is then usually taken to mum for a cuddle before dad and the baby are taken to another room for weighing and first injections.

- Dad then waits for mum in the recovery room for usually 30-40minutes.
- Once mum joins them in recovery, the midwife can help mum breastfeed if mum is feeling well.
- Mum usually stays in recovery for an hour or so for monitoring, and if all is well, your midwife from the ward will receive you and everyone will be transferred to the ward together.
- After transfer to ward both mum and baby will be monitored very frequently for 4-6 hours, then less frequently after that.
- The urinary catheter (tube in your bladder that collects your wee for you) usually stays in until between 6-24 hours depending on the midwife/doctor assessment and hospital policy and ward culture.
- Mum will stay in bed until advised to get up to walk around and/or shower.
- The midwife will help mum feed and change the baby/teach dad for the first day/night.

14: YOUR BODY POST BIRTH

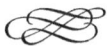

Let me be crystal clear here. **You and your baby come as a package. None of this 'the baby is the only priority' rubbish.**

GENERAL ADVICE FOR ALL MUMS

- I always say that just looking at a hospital can make someone **constipated**. Most women will need the help of laxatives to get them with a poo after birth. Regardless, you want it to be easy when you poo. So start gentle laxatives from day one if you can. Also, order pear juice/prunes/coffee, post birth. (**Yes, you're allowed a coffee** or two post birth! With the baby receiving small amounts of colostrum, caffeine is not likely to go through in any significant amounts. Caffeine is also a

medication we give to premature babies in the nursery to support breathing, so it is not dangerous for them.)
- If they give you laxatives, it'll be super gentle stool softeners in powder or pill form, so don't be afraid of overdoing it.
- If you don't poo by 4-5 days post birth, you'll need additional help to poo with an enema (I.e. Gel up your bottom. So prevention is key here if you want to avoid that).
- **Eat properly.** Don't miss meals. Your body needs energy to make milk.
- **Urinating** will be different the first few days after birth due to all the stretching and pulling in that area. You might not feel like you need to go, or when you go, you might not empty completely. So set alarms on your phone to go every 3-4 hours (or just before a feed) and when you go, go twice. Each hospital will test your ability to wee differently. Some will use Ultrasound, others might measure your wee. They usually do this for your first and/or second wee.
- **Sleep when you can.** Make an afternoon nap your priority. Have dad take the baby for the stroll in the bassinet away from you. For your first baby, you probably won't sleep well while they are in the room with you. You will wake up to every noise they make. You will be up a lot during the night so you MUST sleep during the day.

- **Look after your breasts and nipples** (more on breastfeeding in the next section).
- A belly band can provide great support straight after birth. Most commercial post pregnancy support garments are best used a few days after birth (otherwise it hurts too much) and when you start, only put it on for an hour, then take it off. Gradually wear it for longer periods. This is especially true for caesarean mums.

VAGINAL BIRTH

You will have a heavy period after birth.

- A **shower** morning and night- especially concentrating on your vagina if you have torn or have had a cut (which most women have). If your hospital shower head is removable, give the whole area between your legs a good flush and then pat dry.
- Have your underwear and a pad ready to go and close by so you can put it back on straight away
- An additional shower after you open your bowels (have a poo)
- Please don't miss your **laxatives**
- Make sure your stitches are checked daily
- They can get infected

- The stitches sometimes fall out/come apart too early
- Replace your **perineal ice pack regularly** for the first 3 days
- This reduces swelling and pain
- If you have extensive stitches (with a 3rd of 4th degree tear) do not miss your postnatal physio appointment
- You must manage your bladder and bowel health carefully
- Plan you next birth carefully to avoid this again (use an epi-no, perineal massage or in the case of a 4th degree- consider a caesarean).

Pain relief

- Usually after a vaginal birth you need to ask for pain relief. You'll get some tablets up your bottom after your stitches are done in birth suite and these might last 8ish hours.
- After this you should take paracetamol and an anti-inflammatory regularly (Diclofenac/Ibuprofen), check with your midwife.
- When a doctor prescribes medications, they either make them regular medications (that must be given at certain times) or in a "PRN" or "as needed" section, which means the patient requests/midwife offers it.
- Plenty of women don't need much after a vaginal birth, but a majority of women will

need Paracetamol + anti inflammatory for a couple of days.
- Always check with your doctor before taking anti inflammatories if you have had blood pressure issues in pregnancy (especially with Pre-eclampsia)

CAESAREAN BIRTH

- You will still have a heavy period after birth
- The midwife will check and change your pads after surgery, but once you're out of bed, it's up to you to monitor blood loss.
- **If you're filling up a full pad in one hour, notify a midwife**
- **If you pass a clot bigger than 50c piece, notify a midwife**
- It's normal to lose a bit of blood when you go from lying to standing as blood often pools in your cervix and then releases as you stand
- While you are still in bed, often you will have a drip of fluid and a urinary catheter so you don't have to wee.
- Go slow with eating to begin with.
- **HOT tip**: chew on gum straight after surgery. This has been shown to prevent the occurrence of a complication called a 'paralytic ileus' (where the intestines go into shock after surgery and become paralysed).

- No big lunches/dinner (it'll probably come right back up)
- The midwives/physio will show you how to get in and out and bed. Listen and do it this way every time. Most of your pain will be from getting in and out of bed.
- **Urinate every 3 hours.** If you let your bladder fill up too much, it'll push against your wound and cause more pain. Then as your bladder deflates when you wee it'll hurt again.
- Wound dressings along the caesarean wound are waterproof but can sometimes open up around creased areas. Midwives should check this daily.
- **Pain relief:**
- Paracetamol and an anti-inflammatory (ibuprofen, Diclofenac, Naproxen) are given regularly for your entire stay and should be continued religiously when you go home for up to a week
- Remember to eat with anti-inflammatories
- Your midwives will give these out to you at the hospital, but then it is your job to ask for stronger medication when your pain creeps up
- Endone (oxycodone) or Tramadol are common choices
- They can make you constipated
- Oxycodone can make some people feel dizzy/spaced out
- Once at home, set an alarm to remember its time to take your tablets

- Other medications: most hospitals require women after caesarean to be on a tiny injection of a blood thinner (Clexane, Fragmin or Heparin) once a day to prevent blood clots.
- Movement after surgery
- Technically, as soon as the movement in your legs come back you can get up and stand (usually by 6 hours post birth)
- As soon as your catheter comes out, you'll have to get out of bed every 3-4 hours to wee.
- This time frame is up to you and your team
- Before you get up, make sure you have eaten and have had strong pain relief 30-60mins beforehand.
- The earlier you get up, the better for your recovery. No one was made to stay in bed for 24 or more hours. Get up the same day as your surgery if you can.
- The first 24 hours after your catheter comes out expect to move to the toilet and back, not much more. It might be beneficial to sit in a chair for a bit.
- The next 24 hours, walk around the room, sit in the chair to feed the baby.
- The 3rd day, see if you can go for a slow walk around the ward or just down the corridor. Trust me, by day 3 you need to leave your room for your mental health!
- Don't push yourself too much, you'll pay for it later with pain. But you do need to move your

legs regularly to avoid blood clots in your legs (DVTs).
- Showering after a caesarean
- Use a shower chair but most women find that doing the bending motion to sit down is more trouble than it's worth, so you can just stand.
- Just make sure you don't make the shower too hot and for your first one, not too long.
- You shouldn't need too much help in the shower, I would only request for someone to wipe your legs down as bending the first few days is not fun.

15: THE FOURTH TRIMESTER

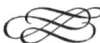

Human babies are born well before they should be.

- We are the only animals that give birth to our young before they can think properly and move around on their own
- This comes down to our big brains and pelvis size, our babies have to be born this early, otherwise they simply wouldn't fit
- Knowing this, you need to treat your baby with this in mind
- Your baby does not know they are separate from you for a good 6 weeks.
- **Expecting them to sleep and function without you is unreasonable**
- So the fourth trimester is this period of transition so the baby can mature
- Skin to skin during the first week with both parents is very beneficial, not only for bonding but also lactation hormones for mum

- Babies like to feel your heart beat, breathing and temperature. It also helps to regulate these things in themselves.
- **Never let a baby younger than 8 weeks cry it out or practice 'controlled crying' this not good for your baby's brain. They do not understand why no one is coming to help them.**

- If your baby is crying, there are only a few reasons at this stage
- Hunger
- Dirty nappy
- Uncomfortable (wind, belly pain, sore head from vacuum delivery, infection)
- Wants cuddles and comfort to know you are there (remember, they don't understand why they are alone).

16: BABY'S FIRST NEEDLES

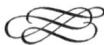

There are only two needles recommended for straight after birth

Babies of this age are given needles into their thighs and recover well straight afterwards.

<u>Vitamin K</u>

- NOT a vaccine
- 1mg of the Vitamin
- No one who has looked at the evidence for this supplement would skip this
- **There is NO evidence of this injection causing cancer or any other disease. The paper that started that rumour was actually made up and false.**
- Prevents life threatening bleeding in baby's brain called Vitamin K deficiency bleeding
- Babies purely breastfeed are at the highest risk
- Surely the natural process of birth does not

require a supplement! Unfortunately, babies are deficient in this vitamin at birth. It helps to clot blood properly.
- There is also an oral version, but it is half as effective and if not given for long enough will not prevent late onset bleeding.
- For full details: https://evidencebasedbirth.com/evidence-for-the-vitamin-k-shot-in-newborns/

Hepatitis B Vaccine

- Babies receive this at birth, 2,4, & 6 months
- The current recommendation is for 4 doses, however at 3 doses the baby can be considered fully immunised to Hep B. This means you can skip the birth dose if you want.
- The birth dose covers babies from 0-2months from getting Hep B so it could be argued that if mum or dad do not have Hep B or are in high risk communities, they don't need it.
- Babies will not get the Hep B dose straight after birth if mum or baby have a temperature or proven infection at birth (at the vaccine can raise their temperature further).

Eye ointment

- Currently required in the US, Canada & many parts of Europe

- Not required in Australia and NZ unless proven infection
- Prevents pink eye caused by Chlamydia and Gonorrhoea (so if you're negative for these infections, do you really need it?)
- Full details: https://evidencebasedbirth.com/is-erythromycin-eye-ointment-always-necessary-for-newborns/

17: BREASTFEEDING

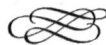

You thought the birth was the HARD part? Ha!

Don't get me wrong, some women breastfeed with the ease of a mother primate.

But those women are few and far between. I mean, have you seen monkey nipples?! They're super long, and their babies are more mature. And so WE, with our immature-should-still-be-in-the-womb-but-can't babies, need to work at this gig.

Look at your nipples. Yes, I mean right now. What do they look like? Are they long, big, short, flat, non-existent or inverted? Nipples come in all sorts of shapes and sizes. How about your breasts? Are they huge, small, have you had a reduction or implants? These are all things that affect breastfeeding and you should tell your midwife about this after birth.

- Crying is a LATE sign of hunger. If a newborn is awake and looking around, chances are they'll want to the feed. Other signs:
- Moving mouth around
- Sticking out tongue
- Sucking on hand/blankie
- Principles of Breastfeeding a newborn
- A baby should feed as soon as possible after birth
- They should feed **8- 12 times in 24 hours** (works out 3-4hourly)
- If he/she cannot latch and feed properly, the mother should express colostrum into a syringe and finger feed the baby.
- Babies need about 1/2 a teaspoon to start with
- We give the baby however much mum can produce. Each mum is different.
- If baby continues to not be able to latch, hand expressing should be done every 3-4 hours plus start an electric breast pump. You need to stimulate your breast for your supply to come in.
- Breasts produce **colostrum** the first three days. It's like a condensed milk for the baby. After day 3, the breasts should start to fill with proper milk. This can be a slow or quick process.
- Principles of latching
- To be fair, every person and their aunty has something to say about this. It's changed across

the years. Just do what works for you. But here are the basic universal principles:
- Baby should be chest to chest
- Place baby's lips next to nipple (they should have to tilt their chin slightly upwards to do this so their nose is clear from the breast once latched)
- **Sandwich your areola** as if you were squishing a hamburger in their mouth (the goal here is to get as much into the baby's mouth as possible.) See videos below.
- Stroke your nipple against lips
- Wait for a wide open mouth
- Bring the baby towards you quickly to get a deep latch
- Make sure the four points of baby's mouth (chin, nose and two cheeks) are all facing the breast evenly. We don't want an uneven angle=uneven latch.
- Let baby establish their latch for ten seconds before you change hand position and get comfortable
- It will hurt for the first few seconds then the pain should go away
- If it continues to hurt (sharp pinchy pain) your latch is shallow and you should de-latch and start again. (De-latch by pushing your finger in between the baby's gums to break the suction. **Never** pull a baby straight off because your baby will take your nipple with him. Yikes!
- **Check your nipple** as soon as the feed finishes.

If it looks squashed in any way, the baby was not deep enough. Keep working on a better latch. It might take a few days or weeks for some people.
- Too many bad latches can lead to nipple grazing/blisters
- **Look after your nipples** by:
- Checking them each feed
- After each feed, hand express one droplet of your milk and coat the nipple. Let it air dry and then put whatever nipple balm you like.
- Most common are just made of plain wool fat: Lansinoh and Marcalan are two popular brands that are safe for the baby.
- If you notice a graze or blister, express on to your nipple between your feeds as well, and it will help them heal faster.
- If you have extensive damage, let your nipples rest for 24 hours and have the baby get expressed breastmilk from a syringe/bottle.
- Breastfeeding is like driving a car, once you've got the skill you have it for life.
- **I highly recommend you get some sort of breastfeeding pillow.**

* **Don't just take my word (or anyone else's) for it. Please go to YouTube and watch some technique videos on how to latch a newborn. Full credit to the amazing mothers and clinicians below:**

There are many different positions to try: https://www.youtube.com/watch?v=7FJuBn2bgNk

Great technique here: https://www.youtube.com/watch?v=41fC0fQs1P8

The lying back method: https://www.youtube.com/watch?v=d8SI4XKkOl8

Disclaimer: Breastfeeding videos with real babies are the BEST way to see how it's done. Keep in mind that although these babies are newborns, they are not a few days old (more like a two-three weeks or more). Newborns in the first few days are often less alert, less likely to open their mouth super wide. They can be lazy/sleepy due to the effects of caesarean drugs, epidurals and other labor drugs. So just keep in mind that you might have a few feeds with a lazy latch or no latch at all.

~

Burping

Bottle-fed babies get more air than breastfed babies, but it's a good habit to burp the babies in between breasts and after a feed. Put baby over your shoulder for 5-10 minutes, patting and rubbing their back. If you don't get air after 10 minutes put them back to sleep.

18: BREASTFEEDING TROUBLES

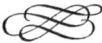

If you are having trouble breastfeeding, remember that it is common to have issues. Be kind to yourself and remember that patience and perseverance can help you do anything in life. I believe in you! And midwives and doctors will support any decision you make as long as you are informed.

Flat/Inverted Nipples:

- I would say that this is the most common cause of babies being unable to latch
- Flat or inverted nipples are a dim a dozen nowadays
- Some babies can latch onto a flat nipple without damage, but most cannot.
- Reason: they just can't get purchase on the breast and slip off, unable to get a latch. The

baby will bob around looking for a nipple that's not there.
- Solution: Active latch with a deep C-hold (really shaping the areola to get the baby to latch. Often a midwife will have to help you do this.)
- If that doesn't work then you will need to express breastmilk and feed by syringe or bottle until your milk is starting to coming so you can use a:
- Nipple shield: a plastic 'nipple' that sticks over your flat nipple to create a shape for the baby to latch on. You will still need to keep expressing once you start using this otherwise supply tends to drop over time.

How to know if baby is getting enough milk:

- Once milk is in, you'll hear gulping and swallowing sounds
- Your breast will go from hard to softer
- Baby is satisfied and sleeps afterward
- Wet nappies and stools are changing colour—black to brown to green (pesto) to yellow by day 5-7 (mustardy).
- If your milk is not in yet (so the first 3 days), you'll need to keep feeding your baby when they ask for it. This will bring your milk in faster.

Oversupply/Engorgement

- Most women having their first baby will have too much milk to start with. Your body needs to learn how much it needs to make.
- You know you have this if your breasts are rock hard (literally) and you are in pain.
- How to deal with it:
- Wake your baby up and have them feed
- Use a heat pack and massage your breast during the feed to help with the flow of milk.
- If after the feed your breasts are still uncomfortable, use a breast pump or hand express for the least possible time (no more than 5 mins) to get rid of more milk
- Don't empty your breast too much as then you are giving your breasts the signal to make more milk. (They slow down milk production when they are full and speed it up when it's empty).

Undersupply

- Make sure a health professional helps you diagnose this. It is easy to misdiagnose yourself. (They will be looking at many things including your breast capacity, weight/growth of the baby etc.)
- Some signs:
- If your baby is dehydrated, loosing weight/not gaining weight despite a solid 8-12 feeds a day and still seems hungry
- Baby is jaundiced

- Baby is lethargic and very sleepy (doesn't have enough energy)
- If your breasts are not getting heavy and full by day 5-7
- How to deal with it:
- After feeding at the breast you pump by hand (if day 1-3) and/or an electric pump.
- By pumping on an empty breast, you give your breasts the signal that they need to make more
- The baby needs to get fed until they are full so after a feed, give the baby as much milk as you can from your expressing plus formula.

Mastitis

- An infection of the breast, usually due to a blocked duct
- **Prevention is key:** get your milk moving, **check them** each feed for lumps of milk. During a feed and in the shower massage them to get them out.
- Symptoms: Hard, red, hot area on breast and flu like feeling.
- How to deal with it: Pull the milk out of the breast by feeding and or pumping. And see your GP **straight away** (do **not** delay this) and get antibiotics. If it's the middle of the night, call an on call doctor or go back to your birth hospital.
- If you are on antibiotics for two days and you

don't see any difference, chances are you need to go back to hospital for IV antibiotics.

Lactation Consultant

- This is a health professional (usually a midwife) who has undergone extensive training and experience to assist women with breastfeeding challenges to feed their baby
- This is the person who will help you if you have breastfeeding issues (latching, under-supply, oversupply, mastitis).
- Most hospitals have one
- You can hire one privately
- Can have different philosophies or ideas on breastfeeding

∼

Do you need a **breast pump**?

- If you have decided to give breastfeeding a good hot go, then you probably will need one.
- You won't use it in hospital (hospital pumps are usually better at stimulation and also you won't have any washing to do).
- Reasons to use one:
- You want to store milk for bottling the baby later
- You have engorgement/too much milk and

need to get rid of some easily to reduce pain in the breast.
- You don't have enough milk and need to stimulate your breasts after the baby has a feed.
- You can't/don't want to latch baby but still want to give breast milk (very common).
- Get an electric one, a hand pump will just give you RSI/wrist problems
- $200 + for a new one
- Can be hired from Hospital or breastfeeding associations
- Can buy second hand from online
- Popular brands: Medela, Avent and anyone that uses a **Spectra** raves about it, however it is a higher end price. (Nothing from this book is sponsored).

There are a lot of great resources for breastfeeding. The following are my HIGHLY recommends. I would rather you watch videos and sign up to Facebook groups than read long essays on the topic:

Dr Jack Newman- Founder of International Breastfeeding Center (lots of videos on his website)

https://ibconline.ca/breastfeeding-videos-english/

https://www.facebook.com/DrJackNewman

Professor Amy Brown- Breastfeeding uncovered

https://professoramybrown.co.uk/articles

https://www.facebook.com/breastfeedinguncovered

The Milk Meg (Lactation Consultant, plenty of info + virtual consults)

https://themilkmeg.com/

https://www.facebook.com/themilkmeg

19: SUPPLEMENTING

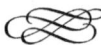

Please note: if you wish to **Formula** feed your baby (exclusively) this is your decision to make and no health professional will question you about it other than to understand you better.

Some women also choose to give colostrum the first few days and then move onto formula after their milk comes in. The most common reason for this is having a bad experience breastfeeding the previous baby. They want their baby to have the benefits of the colostrum but don't want to risk pain/damage of breastfeeding.

I'll tell you what I tell all my ladies. Everyone knows that breastfeeding your baby is best for their health, however, **it is not worth ruining your entire experience of being a mother & ruining your relationship with your baby** and crying every feed to exclusively breastfeed.

If you do not look forward to breastfeeding, fear it, have extensive nipple damage, cry every feed, are in great pain when you feed or simply do not want to do it anymore. **Do not do it.**

Your mother, mother-in-law, sisters, friends do not have to go through this and therefore cannot have an opinion on it. It is your decision.

Cranky midwife rant over.

- There are a few reasons you might need to **supplement**
- This means you give a top up of formula with a syringe or bottle.
- You can also give your breastmilk as a top up in a bottle/syringe if you have enough
- Your midwife will give you an idea of how much — every situation is different.
- Some reasons:
- Loosing excessive weight
- Mum does not have enough milk yet, and the baby is dehydrated/hungry
- Extensive nipple damage or pain during feeding
- Mum has had zero sleep and is too tired to feed any longer
- Baby has dropped blood sugars
- Baby is in the nursery and must take a certain amount per feed

- How to tell if your baby is dehydrated
- Less wet and dirty nappies than expected
- Dry mouth and lips
- Very dry skin
- Always hungry, looking for milk day and night

<u>How to supplement?</u>

- Follow the directions on the back of the formula tin as to how to make it up.
- Make sure your bottles and teats are sterilised by either using a steriliser or submerging them in a saucepan of water and boiling it for 10 minutes.
- Pour the required amount of water into the bottles. Wait 5 mins to cool sightly, then scoop the required scoops in. Wait to cool then put in fridge ready for the next feed.
- I advise you to make up your formula in advance. You can store it for 24 hours.
- When you are ready for your feeds you can easily pour out the required amount out, warm it up by placing the bottle in a cup of hot water and then feeding baby.
- Always check temp of bottle before giving it to baby by squirting a drop onto your wrist.
- For amounts required, ask your midwife or doctor, it goes by the baby's weight. (After 7 days of age it is usually around 150mls per kilo per day for a full feed of formula.)

- If you are doing part breastmilk part bottle, you will need to observe baby's behaviour and see how hungry they are after taking the breastmilk or by going by your midwife or child health nurse's guidelines.

20: THE FIRST 24 HOURS

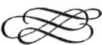

MUM:

- Your job is to rest and recover
- No visitors except your parents- and it must be short
- Don't do a Facebook post if you can help it. Seriously, focus on yourself and getting mental rest for one day at least (especially if you are a sensitive sort of person).
- Write stuff down on your phone, pen and paper, whatever. Get an app to mark down babies feeds and nappy changes. You will be asked this information for many weeks and trust me, no one remembers.
- Don't forget to take your pain killers. If you are not offered them, ask for it.
- If your bottom is super sore, ask the midwives to show you how to feed lying on your side.

- If your catheter has come out: before each feed, go to the toilet for a wee and check your pad.

BABY:

- Baby's job is also to recover
- Babies usually do a big feed straight after birth (they are full of adrenaline) and then do one of two things:
- Either they crash and do a big sleep (most babies do this)
- Or they want to keep feeding
- Babies are made to feed around 3-4 times in the first 24 hours. This is to allow you to rest.
- However, if your baby is being monitored for blood sugar levels, you will need to wake baby up every 3 hours to feed.
- If your baby is less than 2.8kg you should also wake baby up to feed if they've slept more than 4 hours after the start of the last feed.
- Hospital policy and practice differs on this, but generally speaking, you can't overfeed a breastfed baby. (I have seen it happen, but only in the case of a huge supply, not this early).
- Ask the midwife looking after you for advice about when to feed. Generally, I say something like "If the baby hasn't woken up by x'oclock wake them up and remind them."
- Before you feed, wake the baby up.
- You can't just grab a sleeping baby out of the

cot, put it by the nipple and expect them to feed. (I have seen countless people do this).
- You need to wake the baby: Open up their wraps, change the nappy
- Tell the midwife you are about to feed so they can take the baby's observations now (you don't want them to be doing a temperature once you've finished, it'll wake them back up).
- I would generally take this opportunity to do skin-skin. Its great for brain development, bonding and will ensure they stay awake for a proper feed. No, they won't get cold, you actually heat each other up during a feed. NO wraps on top until they are vigorously feeding.
- PRO TIP: If your baby is too sleepy to feed, place them on a flat surface in front of you without anything touching them. Wait a little bit, talk to them, tickle them and they'll start wondering where you are. Grab them back up for the feed.
- **Expected nappies**: 1 wee and 1 black sticky poo minimum
- Plenty of babies often do more
- Some babies take longer to poo than 24 hours, we just need to check that they are able to poo (as in, have a working anus) then just wait for when they are ready.
- Keep the cord out of the nappy if you can, the drier it is, the more quickly it'll fall off (7-10 days, often earlier).
- Your first night is usually a good one, the baby

won't ask you for too much to make sure you get plenty of rest the first day.
- Baby is simple for the first few days:
- Feed them
- Change them
- Cuddle them
- Repeat

21: VISITORS + A WORD ABOUT COVD-19

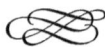

I don't know a single Midwife that loves visitors.

Why? Not because we hate people (I mean, we're midwives, we have to like people- being a midwife or nurse is like a retail job on steroids), it's that visitors make mothers and babies tired.

And if a mother is not tired before her visitors, I can guarantee she will be afterwards.

If COVID-19 taught us anything, was that not having visitors in maternity wards dramatically increased successful breastfeeding rates, increased general happiness of mothers, dads and babies.

Why? Because mothers have time to sleep and rest.

Before this pandemic, on any one day you'd find a woman crying in a maternity ward. Sure, there's hormones abound, but they are so tired they learn why sleep deprivation is used as a torture technique in POW camps.

During COVD-19? I've never seen fewer tears on a maternity ward. And did you know that during the isolation time, premature births decreased? Anyone can see the reason why. Women got to REST + they caught less bugs staying at home.

Visitors who stay for hours during the day forget that this is generally only time for mothers to catch up on sleep.

Visitors who stay for hours interrupt feeds. If there is ever a midwife who got cranky, was because the baby is due to feed, but is delayed because of visitors.

Your baby won't work to your schedule. You'd better get used to it.

Do you know how many times I've walked into a patient's room to have them face timing a relative, for them to say, "The midwife is here, I have to go." And then have them say to me, "Thank god you've come in, we really wanted to get off the call."

Sure, my patients might be being polite to me, but it's happened way too many times for me to believe it's just that. The Fourth trimester is a time for a mother and her baby to rest and recover.

Your body is doing/has done the BIGGEST thing it will EVER do in its lifetime. So why do people need to run around like crazy being productive? Sure, there's stuff to do, but this time doesn't come again for you. Seriously, go lie down for an hour in the afternoon. Cut back on stuff that doesn't NEED to get done right this second.

22: 24-48 HOURS

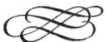

MUM

- For vaginal births: keep icing your bottom, make sure you wee before each feed.
- For C-Section: today is your day to get your catheter up and walk to the toilet. Take it slow, but don't avoid it. Empty your bladder 3-4hourly. Don't overdo the walking.
- Get a rest in during the afternoon because chances are you'll be up most of the night.
- Thought pregnancy swelling was over? Wrong! You'll get a little more swelling after birth in your legs/feet. This is just extra fluid leaving your body. Elevate your legs a couple of times a day to let gravity do its thing. Hospital beds are really useful for this, use it while you have it. Otherwise at home, place a couple of pillow under your feet.
- C-Section mums can also get swelling around

the lower abdomen, around your wound. Usually this is from being in sitting positions for a long. (Let's face it, you're feeding a lot!).
- Learn how to bathe your baby

BABY

- Newborns love to sleep during the day and party ALL night.
- PRO TIP: wake the baby up regularly (if you aren't already) during the day so that they're not starvin' marvin during the night.
- I mean, they'll look like they're starving all night anyway, but if you want your milk to come in, stimulate your breasts with feeds as much as possible.
- If bub will not feed no matter how hard everyone tries, you need to express by hand and give it to them via syringe.
- Remember, I said newborns feed 8-12 times a day? Tonight, your baby will try to do ALL of those feeds.
- If your baby falls asleep on one breast, check their nappy and wake them up to offer the other side.
- Because there is only colostrum in your breasts, it takes a bit of effort for them to get 'full' and even so they get hungry very quickly.
- Feeding hourly is normal at this stage and is called clustering
- When your milk is 'in', this will change as the

baby will get milk drunk after a feed and sleep a little longer. Often at this early stage, you'll feed and put the baby in the cot and they wake up instantly. At milk drunk baby dosen't do this.
- Remember that every baby and every woman is different.
- Each baby has different requirements
- Each woman has a different storage capacity
- Half of the time, your baby simply does not want to sleep on their own and will cry/look for you when you put them down
- Expected nappies: 2 wees and 2 poos (still black/dark)

23: 48-72 HOURS

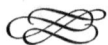

MOTHER

- Vaginal birthers: Keep icing that perineum!
- Caesarean birthers: try to walk a little more today, take the baby for a spin down the corridor. (Wheeling the baby is good because you can use it as a sort of walker)
- Coming up to 72 hours milk should be starting to come in. (For anyone who has not labored before birth, give yourself an extra day for your lactation hormones to kick in).
- Your breasts will start to feel heavier and swollen. Then they'll get hard with milk.
- Blood rushes to your breasts first, and they get swollen, *then* they fill with milk. So you might feel heavy but not be able to express much to begin with.
- Check your breasts each feed for lumps. Lumpiness is a normal part of your milk

coming in, but we don't want lumps to stay in the same spot for too long. So keep an eye for them. When you're in the shower and during feed/expressing, massage those lumps of milk to get them out.
- You can also use heat packs. Heat helps to get the milk moving towards the baby.

BABY

- On the third day, baby's nappies often drop off to completely nothing before they pick up the next day. Your milk should come in soon and rectify this.
- This next night will probably be similar to the previous night with the cluster feeding, so make sure you get an afternoon sleep again.
- If baby is still having trouble latching or has not latched at all, pumping with a breast pump must be done 8 times a day and a Lactation Consultant or senior midwife should give you a plan of action.
- A nipple shield can be introduced if milk is starting to come in or if nipples are every damaged. Depends on the situation.
- If nipples are damaged and it's too painful to latch, resting the nipples for 24 hours and expressing is recommended to allow nipples to rest and heal. After 24 hours, you attempt to latch again.
- Baby's NST (Newborn Screening Test) is due

after 48 hours. This is a universal blood test done on all babies around the world to test for metabolic and genetic in-born diseases. Often done during a feed, baby's heel is pricked and blood is dropped off onto a card and sent to a lab. No news is good news.
- Usually around this time the baby is weighed to check that weight loss is not too much.
- All babies lose weight after birth
- The only babies that gain weight are those with mums who were still breastfeeding their previous baby when they gave birth (so they had a huge supply).
- Most hospitals advise that up to 10 percent weight loss (of birth weight) is acceptable. Anything above ten percent just means that you should review your feeding plan and make sure that milk supply is increasing.
- Some babies will lose a little more before they start to gain.
- They should be back up to their birth weight by 10-14 days post birth

24: 96 HOURS+

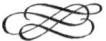

MOTHER

- Vaginal birthers: can still use ice if need be
- C-Section mums: definitely start on that support band/shorts if you haven't already and if you're using a decent amount of strong painkillers, think about cutting back. Sometimes half of pain is the anxiety or expectation of pain rather than pain itself.
- Look after your breasts, watch them, and learn to manage engorgement to avoid mastitis (see Breastfeeding section Ch19)
- You'll start to get into a bit of a routine now, but you should always feed your newborn when they are asking for it, not delaying it because 'its too early'. You can do this with a much older baby, but not anytime soon. try to feed a **hangry** baby, it's not pretty. It's easiest to latch a baby that's awake but not screaming.

BABY

- Once your milk is fully in, baby should be having a nappy every feed. 6-8 wet nappies a day and by now pesto-y green stools (I know, you'll never look at pesto the same way again).
- Start using a nappy cream if you haven't already, a barrier cream (sudocream is really popular). Now you're doing a lot of nappies baby's bum is likely to need it.

25: THE FIRST SIX WEEKS

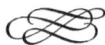

Basic newborn care

- Feed them whenever they want, however much they want (unless you have been advised otherwise in the case of a feeding plan/losing weight)
- Do skin to skin with both parents
- Cuddle and talk and sing as desired
- Keep them clean, dry, and moisturised
- Don't leave them in a dirty nappy
- Use barrier cream for bottom
- Keep cord clean and dry until it falls off (dry after bath)
- Keep eyes clean with water and cotton balls/towel. If sticky- can use breastmilk. If persistently sticky or can't open eye, get checked for conjunctivitis.
- Bath every 2-3 days as needed (you'll have plenty of poo explosions)

- Follow SIDS guidelines for safe sleeping
- Always on back to sleep at the bottom of cot
- No toys or beanies in cot
- No cot bumpers
- Research Co-sleeping. I cannot legally advise you to do this but plenty of people have an opinion. Mothers often do this by accident.
- Tummy time every day as possible
- When baby is awake but settled, allow them time to lie on their tummy to lift their head and look around.
- Go to your weekly weigh-ins with child health or GP
- Thats it! Newborns are simple.

Settling techniques

- Make sure that they are not hungry and have a clean nappy
- Take away from mother (she smells like milk and babies have noses like bloodhounds).
- Walking around with the baby in their bassinet
- Rocking and swaying
- White noise (plenty on YouTube)
- Having baby on their tummy on your lap/chest or in the bassinet while you watch
- Having baby over your shoulder and patting and saying 'shh' or
- singing to them (I've sung many a baby to

sleep- works a treat but use a slow song and sway with it).
- Tight wrapping (not with a sleeping bag)
- Take a video of the midwife showing you how to wrap the baby, there are many different ways to do it. After a week or so a sleeping bag will work. Just remember that babies are used to being in a tight, warm space and too much movement wakes them up/scares them.

26: FOLLOW UP

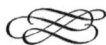

- Make sure you get region specific advice from your hospital before you leave. If you are in a home birthing/midwifery model, check with your midwife, but generally:
- Baby needs to be weighed weekly until 6 weeks. You have three options:
- Home visiting midwife (usually only for the first couple)
- Your GP
- Child Health centre (mothers' groups through here)
- Self-weigh facility at a Pharmacy
- Public
- If you are discharged within 2-3 days in the public system you'll need to see your GP at 7-10 day mark
- You will usually get home care visits from hospital midwives once to twice (during COVID-19 this is via phone or Skype)

- Then you see the government-run Child Health service **weekly** where mothers and babies see a maternal and child health nurse.
- Next vaccines are at 6 weeks with your GP and then follow the vaccine schedule
- Private
- You should get home visits by a hospital midwife or tele health through phone/Skype
- Obstetrician visit 4-6weeks
- Paediatrician visit 4-6 weeks
- Child Health service weekly

Resources for everyone

- Usually in your country there should be a maternal and child nurse help line 24/7
- You should receive a little child health book from the hospital. In this book is not only the record of your baby's immunisations and growth, but also general information about babies and phone help lines.
- In **Australia**
- Pregnancy birth and baby 24/7 phone line - a midwife or maternal nurse to answer your questions 1800 882 436
- The Australian breastfeeding association helpline. These guys have the cheapest breast pumps for rent and 24/7 phone line feeding support for a small annual fee. They also have drop in feeding clinics. 1800 686 268
- Raising Children's Network (website)

- PANDA helpline (perinatal anxiety & depression) 1300 726 306
- **US**
- Check with your hospital/care provider for state specific information
- National Parent Helpline: 1-855-427-2736
- **UK**
- Baby Buddy app
- The association for postnatal illness: 0207 386 0868 (Mon-Fri 10-2pm)
- Tommys.org (answer questions on Instagram and Facebook too)
- Birthtraumaassociation.org.uk
- Pandasfoundation.org.uk

27: BEING AT HOME

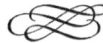

- Do yourself a favour and hire a postnatal doula
- Look some up in your area and see what packages they offer and what they do (usually things like meals, massages, special postnatal herbal mixtures, help with feeding, settling and caring for you and your baby.
- Most cultures did this for women post birth automatically, I think it's a shame we don't care for our new mothers like this anymore.
- Or if that's not your vibe, at least a cleaner or someone to do your meals
- You can also use your mum, but some people are not in a position to have/want their mum/in laws stay with them
- Try and get into a routine
- Feed the baby, change nappy, back to bed
- Bath (every second night)
- If you want a good milksupply get three square

meals and drink 2-3L of water daily. Don't muck around with this. Your body is using up calories to make milk. If you're a normal weight and anybody has the nerve to tell you to watch your weight/body/calories right now, give me their number and I'll tell them what's what. Seriously. I don't have time for that. No one should.

- Please don't feed your newborn baby when they are lying flat in the cot/crib/couch. They can choke. And it's bad for your back. (I have seen people do this with both breast and bottle).

28: YOUR NEXT BABY

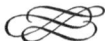

You can get pregnant again very quickly

I have seen women coming back to their six week check pregnant again.

Please use contraception!

You can have sex again pretty soon after birth (I mean, this is why we always knock on doors loudly before we enter— just joking! I mean no I'm not; I know a midwife or two that has walked in on an awkward situation.) But seriously, tell your partner to wait. If you're having trouble with this use the following pre prepared responses:

1. I've just had major abdominal surgery. Get off me.

2. My stitches are not healed I could get an infection and then you wouldn't be allowed there ever again. It'll be the turkey baster for the next baby.

I mean, who would ask questions after that?

I'm hoping you'll both be so tired either of you can't think of anything else. If all else fails, tell him he's allowed to watch the football as long as he wants this weekend.

～

Your perineum takes roughly 2 weeks to heal for a regular injury. You **do not** want an infection there, trust me.

～

Your uterus takes 6 weeks to get back into your pelvis to its normal size. You can feel your uterus straight after birth at your belly button level. Then it goes down a little every day. It takes a full 1 year for your uterus to regain its nutrients and take stock of its life. Give it one year of rest if you can. It's worked hard, geez.

If you've had a c-section you seriously want your scar to heal before you go stretching it again with another baby. Two years for this one, please.

29: THE MOST IMPORTANT TIPS

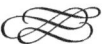

In general:

- Do your research
- Know your birthing and care options with your care provider
- "Blessed are the flexible, for they do not break." (In other words, be flexible)
- Trust your gut/instincts
- Don't worry about what other people think and focus on yourself and your family
- Attend to your self care daily (and talk with your partner about how you can do this)
- Communicate your needs and wants to your partner
- Make a plan for your mental health post having the baby
- Learn how to set boundaries with other family and friends

More specifically:

- Know that you can and should change your health care provider if you are not comfortable with them or their methods or 'vibe' (be it an obstetrician, midwife or paediatrician).
- Write a flexible birthing plan
- Understand what newborns need (food, nappy change, cuddles cuddles and more cuddles)
- Learn about your baby's psychology and what they need at each age group
- WASH YOUR HANDS. After a nappy, before you breastfeed, BEFORE and after you go to the toilet
- Watch Breastfeeding videos on YouTube (if you intend to breastfeed)
- Get an app to log your feeds and nappies. If it's your first baby, you need to do this you can't trust your memory.

AFTERWORD

And that's it from me!

If you enjoyed reading this or found it helpful please leave a review. That's the biggest thing I need to spread this information around.

If you have an comments, questions, or recommendations, let me know at pissedoffmidwife.com.

Sign up to my newsletter for more tips and interesting facts about childbirth.

I'm also planning a series for student midwives coming soon.

Thank you and have a great day!

www.ingramcontent.com/pod-product-compliance
Lightning Source LLC
Chambersburg PA
CBHW050319010526
44107CB00055B/2305